RELEASED!

Healing Through Bi-Polar

Katrina A. Campbell

Released! Healing Through Bi-Polar
© 2016 by Katrina Campbell

ISBN-13: 978-1530686698

ISBN-10: 1530686695

Printed in the USA via CreateSpace

http://tiny.cc/Released

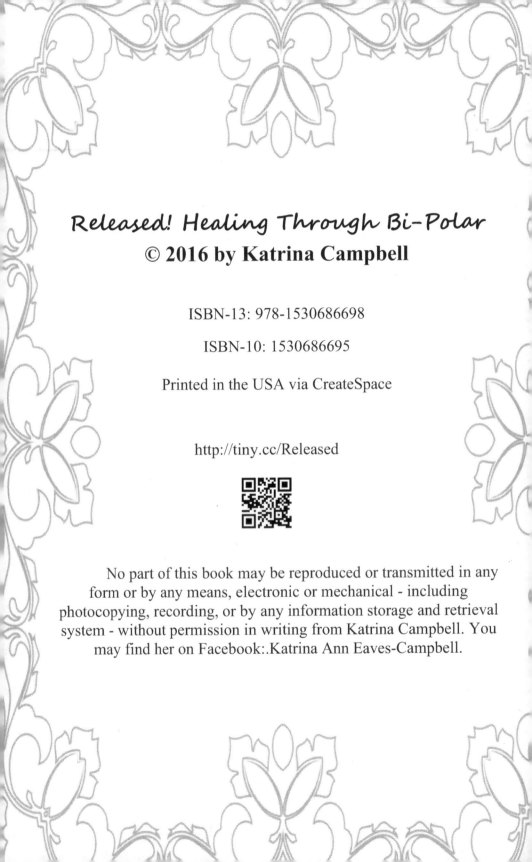

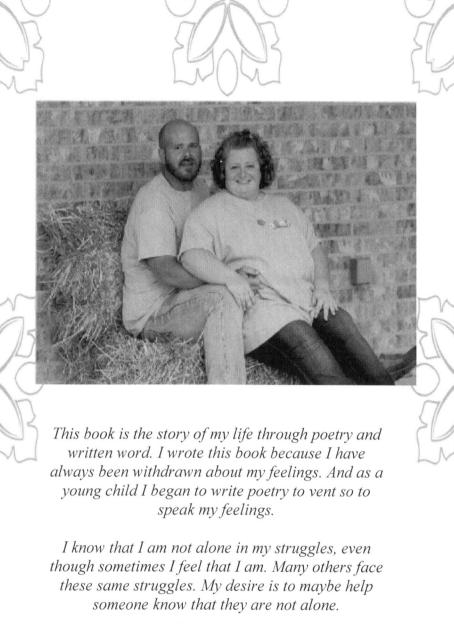

This book is the story of my life through poetry and written word. I wrote this book because I have always been withdrawn about my feelings. And as a young child I began to write poetry to vent so to speak my feelings.

I know that I am not alone in my struggles, even though sometimes I feel that I am. Many others face these same struggles. My desire is to maybe help someone know that they are not alone.

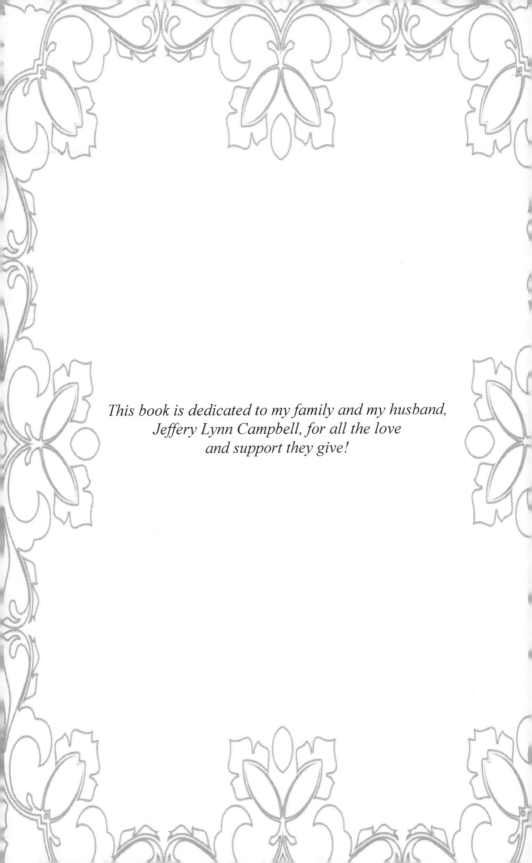

This book is dedicated to my family and my husband,
Jeffery Lynn Campbell, for all the love
and support they give!

One week ago today I did my final packing, loved on my kitties- Figaro, Sampson, Daisy, and dog Lewis, took one last look at my trailer (which I didn't realize how much I loved it until that very moment) and I headed out the door. My folks were taking me to Little Rock, Arkansas where my sister and her family lived.

While Teresa's house was on the agenda it was by no means my destination. Everything I knew was about to change. Well all except one thing and that one thing was God. He is the same yesterday, today and forever! Glory to His name!

I was now residing at a place called the Dorcas House which is a safe haven as well as a battle ground for woman who have been abused and beaten or are struggling to overcome addiction.

And then there are those like me who came with both.

What I have discovered is that abuse and addiction like to embrace each other and when they do life becomes hopeless. I am here because I attempted suicide just 4 weeks ago. My family decided that I could not live on my own any longer and that I needed some real help.

I came from a good, upright standing family. A family that instructed and disciplined my sister and me in the ways of the Lord. I know right now some of you are thinking; okay so what does this chick have to tell me that I haven't heard before? And the truth is…maybe nothing, but I pray that as you read that you will find comfort in my pain. Peace because of my sorrow. All while taking to heart that you are NOT ALONE!

So here's my start. I was born in Quincy, Illinois on October 16, 1975. My dad was a Pastor of a small church in a town called Warsaw, Right on the Mississippi River. I don't think we lived there long, but that was my beginning:

a tiny, sickly child, one who was allergic to milk, full of worms and from what I've been told very unlovable yet needy.

Now my dad was and is also very sickly. And at a young age my sister and I were separated from our folks for a spell while momma took care of daddy while he was in the hospital.

My sister and I stayed with some relatives during this time. Life's tragedies really began here. I was abused by a family member who I love and still care very much about. Neither names nor details are necessary, for these things are covered by the Blood of Christ.

Growing up…the first 7 years I remember moving three times, until we finally ended up in Grand Rapids, Michigan. And it was there we stayed until just two years ago. We moved to Missouri when I was 33.

Oh no, I'm jumping the gun here. Let's go back to when I was 7 and we were settling in our new home in Grand Rapids. Everything was different, the schools were bigger, the tea wasn't sweet, and the people, well they sure talked funny! Them Yankees!

The abuse by that family member came out and my family struggled with how to handle the pain that it had caused in me and now in the rest of my family. Some years went by and now by the time I was 13, the spirit of rebellion had already attached its self to me. I was naughty and withdrawn. Depression set in. My thoughts were dark and so was my heart.

Fight for Life

Another year another day
It doesn't matter what I say
I'm too scared to know why;
The only thing I know is that I want to die.
One on one they fight determined to crucify.
People come to watch me die
They stand and watch my blood and laugh as
my veins run dry.
I get up and wipe away my tears;
Knowing that tomorrow I will have new fears.
I see a hand in front of me.
It's reaching as to help.
As I put my hand forward;
I see a door ahead, straight and onward.
Now I have a friend, he's my helping hand.
He travels with me as I walk this land.
I turn my head and my friend is gone.
The crowds are back, the fighting carries on.
Eating at my heart
Poking at my eyes, these people won't stop until I am dead.
Lying peacefully upon my crystal bed.
I shut my eyes,
Praying I go to heaven in the skies.

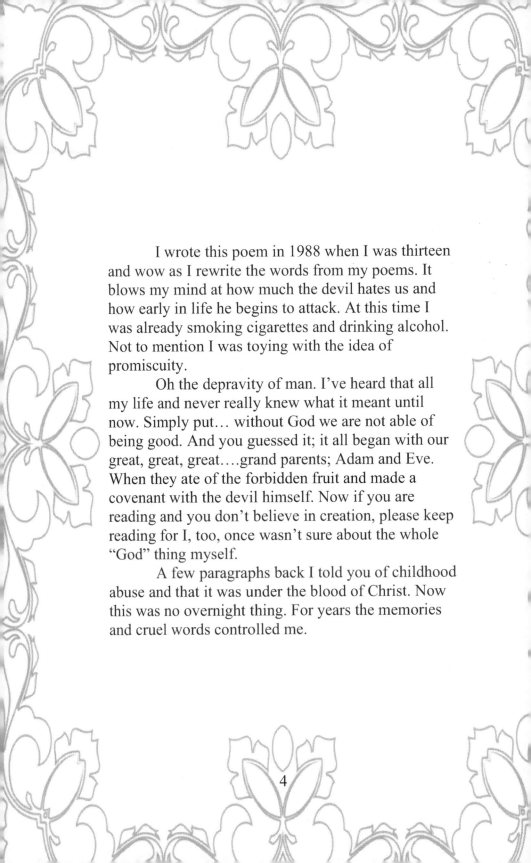

I wrote this poem in 1988 when I was thirteen and wow as I rewrite the words from my poems. It blows my mind at how much the devil hates us and how early in life he begins to attack. At this time I was already smoking cigarettes and drinking alcohol. Not to mention I was toying with the idea of promiscuity.

Oh the depravity of man. I've heard that all my life and never really knew what it meant until now. Simply put… without God we are not able of being good. And you guessed it; it all began with our great, great, great….grand parents; Adam and Eve. When they ate of the forbidden fruit and made a covenant with the devil himself. Now if you are reading and you don't believe in creation, please keep reading for I, too, once wasn't sure about the whole "God" thing myself.

A few paragraphs back I told you of childhood abuse and that it was under the blood of Christ. Now this was no overnight thing. For years the memories and cruel words controlled me.

To Return

Back to blackness
Return to cold
Remembering yesterday
Recalling the old

Hating my childhood
Feeling lost in distress
I grew up when he tore my first dress.

He has stolen from me my childhood,
I remember feeling afraid.
I was stripped of all humanity,
But I loved him so I obeyed.

To return...
Would be a nightmare
Going back would bring more shame.
For deep inside I feel that I am to blame.

I want to be a kid, I grew up to fast
I was too busy praying for a better future,
Never looking on the past.

It torments me now, it won't go away
Deep inside I live the pain of yesterday.

I think letting go of hurt, hurts more than the hurt itself. We somehow make it our identity. And you know what, it's not who we are at all, rather it is something that has happened to us. So stop living that lie, you are not a whore! Rather you can be made whole!

The Bible says that he who the Son sets free is free indeed! Let it go, as a former pastor of mine says, "Go to Lowes , get a ladder and get over it!"

Please know that I am not trying to be insensitive, as truly I have felt your pain and it is because I have felt your pain that I say to you, let go, forgive your abuser, your attacker and even yourself.

Even though I was raised with this knowledge of freedom and peace, it took me 35 years and a lot of garbage to figure it out. And even though I was raised with this truth, knowing that God does has a plan for me, for each of us. (Jeremiah 29:11) I still wondered. I felt so dirty and worthless.

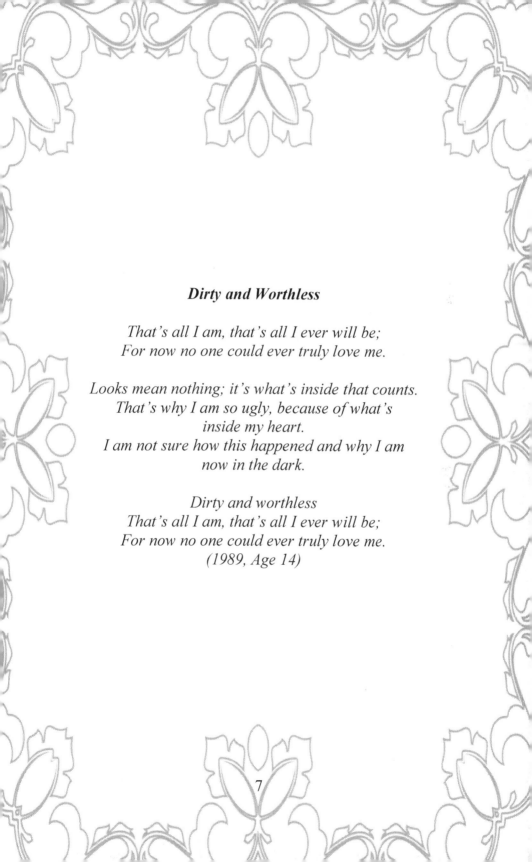

Dirty and Worthless

That's all I am, that's all I ever will be;
For now no one could ever truly love me.

Looks mean nothing; it's what's inside that counts.
That's why I am so ugly, because of what's
inside my heart.
I am not sure how this happened and why I am
now in the dark.

Dirty and worthless
That's all I am, that's all I ever will be;
For now no one could ever truly love me.
(1989, Age 14)

This next poem I'm fixing to share with you I also wrote when I was 12. You may be wondering how such a young person can be so sad. I've wondered that too. You see the devil is a thief; he comes to steal, kill and destroy. He is after the heart of every girl and every boy. Feeling alone and lost is all I knew. Does this ring a bell with you?

Inside My Shirt

Heart ache after heart ache, tear after tear.
Losing all love is my greatest fear.
When friends fight, and schools going wrong
I fell like I do not belong.

Have you ever felt this sadness and sorrow?
I have no peace; I know things will go
wrong again tomorrow.

Slowly dying away,
I face this anger nearly every day.
Sorrow after sorrow, hurt after hurt.
I feel my heart dying inside my shirt.

I hate to be sad, I don't like being down.
But sometimes I feel as if I'm not wanted around
I know that people love, that's common sense.
But inside my heart I'm feeling lonely and tense.

Heart ache after heart ache, tear after tear.
Losing all love is my greatest fear.
Sorrow after sorrow, hurt after hurt.
I feel my heart dying inside my shirt.
(1987, Age 12)

Locked Up

Locked up in a room
I fell so alone
Locked up in a room
It's like my own death zone
Four walls surround me
There's not even a door
Just the wall, a ceiling and the floor
Here are the tears of pain
In this room lie my tears of sorrow
I will be in this room again tomorrow
Locked up in this room
It's locked up so tight
Locked up in a room
Here alone I fight
It is all too familiar, it is all so old
This room is so empty lonely and cold
Locked up in this room
I'm waiting for my time
Locked up in this room
I hate this life of mine
Locked up in this room
I wish the world would end
Locked up
Here in this room, I'm my only friend.
I just kept on living day to day.
Not having any hope of being or feeling different.

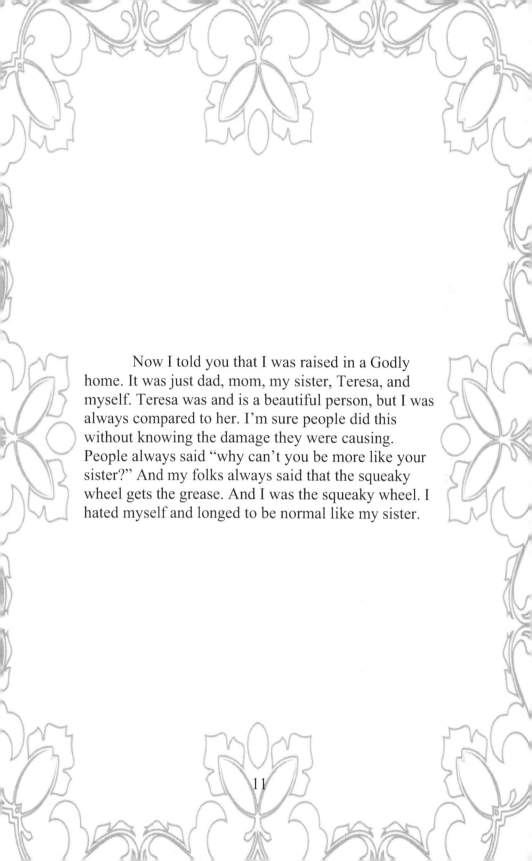

Now I told you that I was raised in a Godly home. It was just dad, mom, my sister, Teresa, and myself. Teresa was and is a beautiful person, but I was always compared to her. I'm sure people did this without knowing the damage they were causing. People always said "why can't you be more like your sister?" And my folks always said that the squeaky wheel gets the grease. And I was the squeaky wheel. I hated myself and longed to be normal like my sister.

I Hate Myself

Always screwing up
Looking very dumb
Cutting on my wrists
Wishing I was numb

I don't like living, but,
I am afraid of dying.
So sick of failing,
Why keep trying?

I hate myself,
And everything I do.
I hate myself,
I wish I was like you.

I can't do anything right.
Sick of crying every night.
Lying in my bed,
Gun pointing to my head.

Why am I so stupid?
I'm so tired of feeling afraid
I guess I get what I deserve.
What a terrible price I've paid.

I hate myself,
And everything I do.
I hate myself,
I wish I was like you.
(1994)

So now that you know I struggled with jealousy and insecurity. Perhaps you will be pleased to know that God says we are all fearfully and wonderfully made. Psalms 139:14 So, while Teresa may have been and still is better than some things as me; it does not mean that she is better. Just different!

Please don't compare yourselves to others. God doesn't. It took me a long time to realize the the Great I Am made me who I am.

Try

Try, try, try
That's all I ever do.
Sometimes I give up,
Especially when I am blue

Try, try, try
I'm trying for you.
You cut me like a knife.
Here I go wrecking my life

Try, try, try
I will never give up
Because trying's what I do.
Try, try, try
I'm tired, aren't you?
(1991)

So here I am a teenager. I was diagnosed with manic depression, which today is known as Bi-Polar. My life was on a downward spiral. And to make matters worse I was finally of the age that my parents said I was old enough to date. Oh sweet 16!

Really there was nothing sweet about it except Alan (I'm calling him this for privacy reasons). He was my first love. He was kind and caring, brave and loyal. We were together 5 years. I don't know how he dealt with me. Just 1 and ½ years after we started to date I attempted to kill myself. I felt so unworthy of love.

I Close the Door

All this time I thought it was you hurting me,
Now I realize it was me hurting you.
Well I am sorry for that; I guess I didn't know I was wrong.
I'll fix it now, for,
Here is where I don't belong.

I've been so selfish, I've been so blind.
Once I die, only the happy will be left behind.

I wish I could be normal and I wish I could stay.
But unfortunately
I am f@#$ed up and can't keep destroying life's this way.
I am sorry if this hurts you, it will be better in the end.
All this time you trusted me, when I wasn't a real friend.

I won't hurt anyone anymore,
The last chapter of my life.
So good bye, I close the door.
(1992)

That was my suicide note, God spared me because He had much more in mind!

Alan stayed right by side while I was in the hospital. He was a good young man, faithful and true. While I was mean and cheated on him with numerous people. So let's see, 17 years old drinking, smoking, and sex was my style. Still lost in depression, life went on. I was hearing voices and seeing things, this became my new reality, I fought it.

No

No, I am not going to let this happen.
I won't let it destroy my everything.
No, how can I stop this; why does it burn?
Why does it sting?
Not this time I say.
Not this time, at least I hope and pray.
Crazy, crazy, crazy
Take away your darkness and you haunting tone.
Please I beg, please leave me alone.
No more voices
No more fear
Please let go, I wanting to be near.
Near to someone.
Tear down theses walls.
Can't you hear my lonely calls?
I'm so close, but so far away.
No, no, no not today.

Betrayal Inside

I am really quite tires of this betrayal I fell inside
I keep looking for a shelter, but find I have no place to hide
Overwhelmed at times yes, I am miserable at times too
It seems that lately I'm always feeling depressed or blue
Every friend I have leaves me
Every companion leads me astray.
I hate you damn people who make me feel this way.

I trust in those I shouldn't,
Seek love from those who couldn't.
Many times I have been stabbed in the back,
It seems those so called friends are always ready to attack

No one ever understands
People are constantly making demands.
Their demanding trust, demanding care.
Demanding that I must always be there.
I give of myself always, why do they treat me like they do?
Don't they realize I am human and I have feelings too?

Friends and family have both rejected me
I guess I cannot see the way others see.
I would never want to betray a trust a trust
I've done that before, and I'll never do it again

Why can't they help me?
Do they want to help me?
No, I think not.
Everyone in this world is a selfish little snot!
Only thinking of them and trying to get ahead.
Always wanting to win, not caring if it
leaves someone dead.

I don't like hurting people, I know what it's like to hurt.

It frightens me to think about becoming one of them.
One of those people whose future looks so dim
Aren't those people lonely, I sure know I am.
I am a true friend to many, but none are true to me.
Should I become what I would really hate to be?

While making bad choices I was working at Wendy's and meet some "friends". I was going to parties and trying to fill the void in my heart with worldly things. I was raped. Still doing the wrong thing and putting myself in bad places I was raped again. Not saying these occurrences were my fault, but I did make the choice to be at those wrong places. So, in dealing with this I just wanted to die even more.

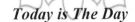

Today is The Day

Today is the day that I want to die.
It seems as if every time I talk;
Every sentence ends with a sigh.
Not knowing what to say, and not knowing what to do.
The people who love me, well they are getting few.

No one understands.
No one seems to care.

They fuss and fight, and tell me what to do.
They only see things from their point of view.

How I want to die.
How I hate to live.
People act as if I should always give.
Give more of myself than I have to offer.
I'm to look in the face of my every scoffer.

I'm to show hate to the ones who've hurt me,
And anger to those I hate.
Rage to the ones who've used me.
This means,
I would truly hate myself.
For at myself I am most angry with.

Today is the day that I want to die.
It seems as if every time I talk;
Every sentence ends with a sigh.
Not knowing what to say, and not knowing what to do.
The people who love me, well they are getting few.

Sometimes

Sometimes I want to cry
Deep inside I feel to die
I feel to scream
I wish to fight
Holding my pain in oh so tight
The pain is growing I can't take much more.
My heart is already trampled on the floor.
So many feelings, with no one to confide.
I can't cry lately, it's as if my heart has died.
I know the hiding my feeling isn't great
For inside of me grows anger and hate.
Sometimes when I am alone I cry, but my
feeling I can't show.
For my heart must no one ever know?

Alan finally broke up with me after I had completely broken his heart. Next I'm in my twenty's. Add smoking Marijuana to the mix. I was at the bar nearly every night. One night stands, stealing, lying and just plain living only for myself. I tried to tell myself that I was better off and that Alan never really loved me.

So Long

I can't believe it's been so long since I've kissed you.
I can still remember the warmth of your lips, to
the point of touch.
I can still feel your arms around my body,
holding me close-
Dear God, why do I miss you so much?

Where did you go?
Why did you leave?
Time has not erased my love for you
Nor has separation made me forget
You are still as fresh in my mind as the spring breeze.

And if it was so long ago, why do I still
hurt like it was yesterday?
Tell me, if it's been so long then why does my
heart feel the same?
Memories of you still fill my head;
To this day you are the first thing on my mind
when I crawl out of bed.

Even though it's been so long, I still love you.

Go On

Go on with life; please quit living in the past.
He's gone, he left you, so turn and walk away.
True love is knocking on your door today.

Go on, it's over; it's not your fault
Quit beating yourself- stop with the constant assault.

Learning to love again will be hard, but worth it.
Take a chance and you will find love can be perfect.
Open the door, tear down the wall.
Answer true love, because it calls.

It's over, let it be over.
Go on.

Remember How to Forget

At times I find myself missing the old days.
The way we use to laugh and the way we use to play.
The way we danced, and our little walks.
Our so unimportant arguments and all night long talks.
I remember it like it was yesterday.

I know that times have changed,
It took so long for my life to get rearranged.
But I am glad you are not with me;
And I am glad that we don't share;
All the things we use too.

It's not that I have stopped caring,
It's all about moving on.
Why live in yesterday, when it's gone,
Long gone.

Can you still see my smile?
Just as I can feel your warm embrace?
If given time, all these memories will be erased.

It may hurt now, but it will not hurt forever.
A time will come when you will see it's for the better.
It's okay to remember, and it's okay to cry.
Just don't carry the hurt with you, and
remember how to forget.
(02-14-1996)

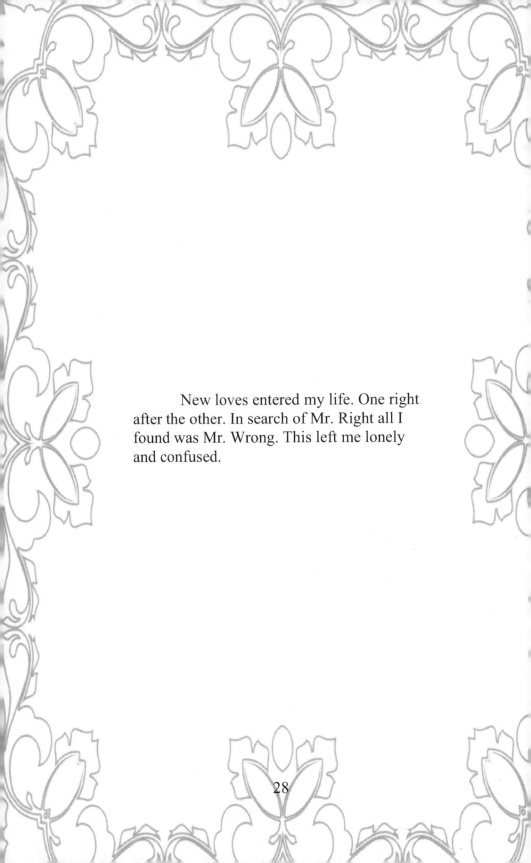

New loves entered my life. One right
after the other. In search of Mr. Right all I
found was Mr. Wrong. This left me lonely
and confused.

Confused Heart

Lonely, Cold, Sad and blue
That's how I feel when you treat me like you do.

Why can't you leave me?
Why do you care?
You always hurt me, I feel lost in despair.

I hate you, but, I love you; please let me go.
How much you hurt me, I guess you'll never know.

Lost, Loved, feeling low and down.
If I bottled all my tears from you, I'd drown.

I'm so lost without, I can't live without you, but,
I wish you would go away.
I'm sick of hurting, and I want to stop feeling this way.

Confused and hopeless, I feel so lost.
If I could I'd change no matter what the cost.

I'd give my life, my heart, my soul.
I'd give anything to feel loved and whole.

Why do you control? Just let me be,
But please don't ever stop loving me!

We belong together, we should be apart.
These are the feelings from my confused heart.

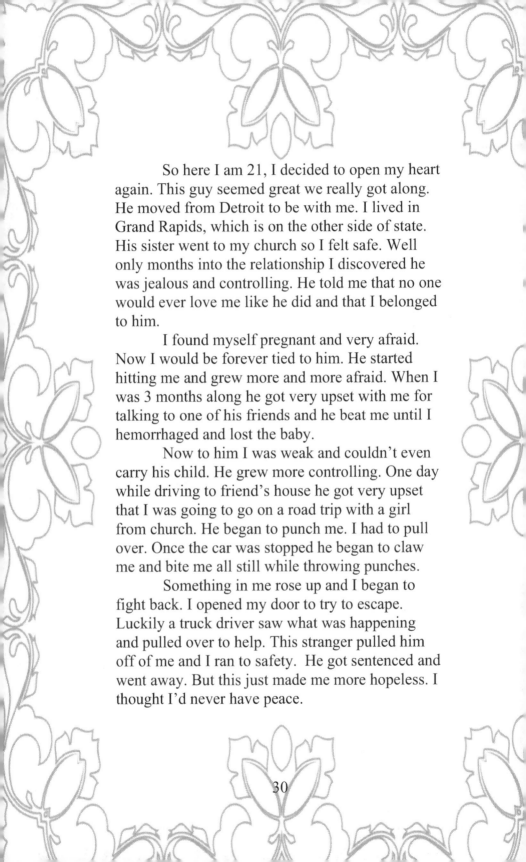

So here I am 21, I decided to open my heart again. This guy seemed great we really got along. He moved from Detroit to be with me. I lived in Grand Rapids, which is on the other side of state. His sister went to my church so I felt safe. Well only months into the relationship I discovered he was jealous and controlling. He told me that no one would ever love me like he did and that I belonged to him.

I found myself pregnant and very afraid. Now I would be forever tied to him. He started hitting me and grew more and more afraid. When I was 3 months along he got very upset with me for talking to one of his friends and he beat me until I hemorrhaged and lost the baby.

Now to him I was weak and couldn't even carry his child. He grew more controlling. One day while driving to friend's house he got very upset that I was going to go on a road trip with a girl from church. He began to punch me. I had to pull over. Once the car was stopped he began to claw me and bite me all still while throwing punches.

Something in me rose up and I began to fight back. I opened my door to try to escape. Luckily a truck driver saw what was happening and pulled over to help. This stranger pulled him off of me and I ran to safety. He got sentenced and went away. But this just made me more hopeless. I thought I'd never have peace.

Forever, Never, Returning

It's been forever that I have felt this way.
Never have I breathed peace for more than one day.
Returning always to the nightmares and closed in walls.
Forever going back to those haunting calls.
Never can I go home again;
Returning wouldn't be the same.
Forever I will be locked up in screwed up brain.
Never can I seem to find the light.
Returning to sleeplessness every single night.
Forever searching,
Never will I be free of my pain.
Returning daily, stuck in the same old rain.
I shall be forever, never, returning

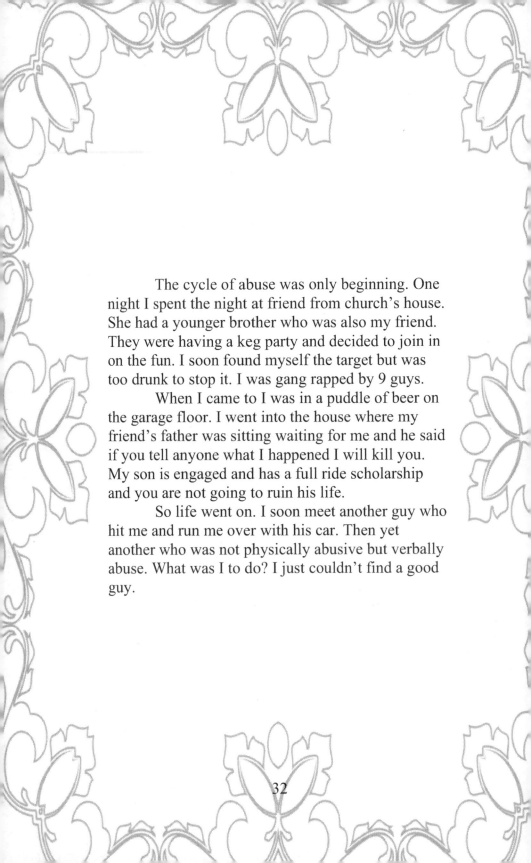

The cycle of abuse was only beginning. One night I spent the night at friend from church's house. She had a younger brother who was also my friend. They were having a keg party and decided to join in on the fun. I soon found myself the target but was too drunk to stop it. I was gang rapped by 9 guys.

When I came to I was in a puddle of beer on the garage floor. I went into the house where my friend's father was sitting waiting for me and he said if you tell anyone what I happened I will kill you. My son is engaged and has a full ride scholarship and you are not going to ruin his life.

So life went on. I soon meet another guy who hit me and run me over with his car. Then yet another who was not physically abusive but verbally abuse. What was I to do? I just couldn't find a good guy.

Crying Wolf

I've been crying wolf
I have been telling lies
Hiding my thoughts and
Living in diskies.
I use to cry wolf, now,
I just cry.

Now when I need someone, here alone I die.
I pushed people away, and I drew people in,
But only to lie; no one really knows who I am
I lock them out, I let them,
But only to slam the door shut again.

I'm alone; I have nothing because I change so oftenly.
Can people ever love, love the real me?
I never should have lied,
If I was truthful, my heart might not have died.
I live a lie, and I forgot the truth.
My life is lost; it drowned in the pain of my youth.

I have been crying wolf
I have been telling lies
Hiding my thoughts and
Living a disguise
I use to cry wolf, now,
I just cry.

All Alone Again

It seemed so right, it seemed so real.
Now how am I supposed to feel?
You said you want to slow down,
But how when we are already stopped.

I never should have weakened,
I should not have given in,
For now I find myself alone again...

They come and they go, but never to stay.
I thought that changed when I meet you,
But I see you leaving, another run a way.

It feels good for a while, living in love...
Actually living in denial.
You left me, put me through pain.
So here I am...
All alone again.

So now I'm 27 years old. Finally moving out of Mom and Dad's house. I was living with a man, dealing drugs and still drinking nearly every day.

At this point in my life I told God to "screw off" and that I was finally free of religion and all its chains. I was living for me! At least that's what I thought. I was actually living for the devil, doing his work and not even realizing it.

One day while cleaning my house and jamming to some Metallica. I felt the absence of God. You see growing up He was present in our home protecting us and giving us peace, but now, He wasn't there! In an audible voice I heard God say" This is the last time I'm going to call you."

That really got a grip on me. You see it wasn't that He was giving up on me it was that my heart was becoming so hard that I wouldn't be able to hear Him again. Right then and there I gave my heart to Christ. Broke up with the current guy and got a place of my own.

I quit drinking, threw away most of my cd's and even gave away my Play Station, as I wanted to give my time to God. My outlook on life changed!

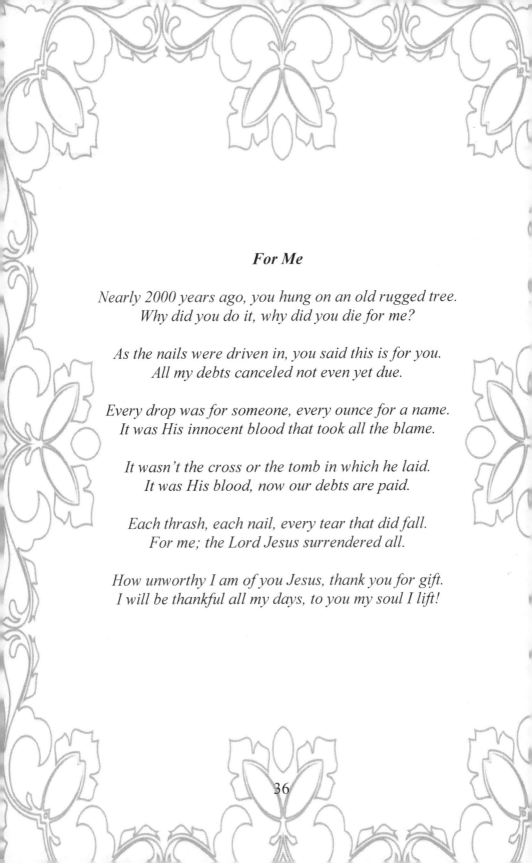

For Me

Nearly 2000 years ago, you hung on an old rugged tree.
Why did you do it, why did you die for me?

As the nails were driven in, you said this is for you.
All my debts canceled not even yet due.

Every drop was for someone, every ounce for a name.
It was His innocent blood that took all the blame.

It wasn't the cross or the tomb in which he laid.
It was His blood, now our debts are paid.

Each thrash, each nail, every tear that did fall.
For me; the Lord Jesus surrendered all.

How unworthy I am of you Jesus, thank you for gift.
I will be thankful all my days, to you my soul I lift!

I gained a new respect for my mom and dad. I saw them in a different light. My mom and I always had a good relationship but my dad and I were different and couldn't see eye to eye. But God was working on that.

A Woman Who Fears the Lord

Loving, patient; kind yet stern.
From you mom, these are the things I learned.

I always knew you loved me, but never understood why.
All I knew is that you were there for me
hearing my every cry.
You gave your love unconditionally,
Like Christ because that's how it's supposed to be.

Many nights you would stay awake and pray;
That under the Lord's shadow I would stay.

Every heartache, every tear…
As you once said; you tethered me to the cross by prayer.

I know God trusted you, to give you a mess like me.
Because of your example, in Christ I am free.

I now know why the bible says," A woman who fears the
Lord is to be praised."
If you had not feared, loved and served our
Savior I would be lost.
Like Him, you gave your life for me not caring the cost.

So thank you mom, for serving Jesus and
teaching me the way.
Because of you I am the woman of integrity
you see today!

She is clothed
She is clothed with strength and dignity;
She can laugh at the days to come.

Proverbs 31:26 she speaks with wisdom,
And faithful instruction is on her tongue.

Proverbs 31:30 Charm is deceptive, and beauty is
fleeting;
But a woman who fears the LORD is to be praised.

Thank you mom for feeding me sheltering and
teaching me the way.
I'm still learning from you. I learn from you every day.
To be raised in a Godly home was the key of my Salvation.
You gave me something to stand on, Gods sure
foundation.
Having turned my back on what I knew,
You where faithful praying I would come
back to what is true.
While I been serving the lord six years, and
you've been my mom for 32.
I am amazed and at beauty and love I find in you.
Going through the beatitudes and seeing what they mean.
You give light to all by whom you are seen.
You are anointed and obedient. Strong and true.
Big must that heart be, that's beats inside of you.

The Hummingbird

Today I saw a humming bird
It hovered near and stayed
As if a gift from you so lovingly displayed.
It ate of nectar as I eat of your bread
You love me is what I heard said
It stayed so close and had no fear,
A lovely picture you painted for me, I will
forever hold dear
To some it may be just a hummingbird, but I
see it as a gift
You alone oh lord my soul do I lift
Being made in his image,
When it looked at me, did it see its creator face?
Its wings its body so intricately placed
Look around you today and take in all that
he has done.
Not only does he give us gifts like the hummingbird,
he gave us his son
Be thankful for all the little these that he
so freely gives.
Now take up his yoke dear children and live, live, live.

Stages of a Mother

At first you were a mommy, because that's all
I could say.
I learned to love you as you rocked me each day.

Next you were a mom, I had begun to grow.
Trying to do things that you said had to be so, so.

Then I had an attitude. I won't say what I
thought you were.
But you were always there for me, that
much is for sure.

Now you are a mother, because I have learned
respect with fear.
I hold you highly mother, you are so dear.

We have a love like no other kind.
That's love is in our hearts, our souls and our mind.

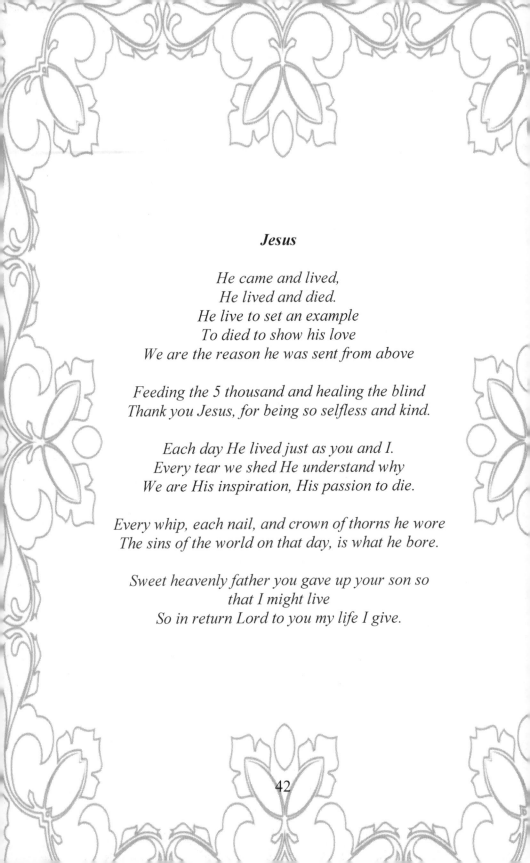

Jesus

He came and lived,
He lived and died.
He live to set an example
To died to show his love
We are the reason he was sent from above

Feeding the 5 thousand and healing the blind
Thank you Jesus, for being so selfless and kind.

Each day He lived just as you and I.
Every tear we shed He understand why
We are His inspiration, His passion to die.

Every whip, each nail, and crown of thorns he wore
The sins of the world on that day, is what he bore.

Sweet heavenly father you gave up your son so
that I might live
So in return Lord to you my life I give.

Mighty Messiah

My life has been crazy, often full of pain.
What I counted as lost, now I count for gain.

Things happen and people go away,
But Jesus loves me and He will never stray!

He calms me sometimes as He did the sea,
He is faithful and He'll do for you as he has done for me.

He holds my hand so tightly when I need His
strength and love
He is the Mighty Messiah, but yet as gentle as a dove.

He has told us over and over His love will never fail.
In Jesus we have the victory, so let His light prevail!

For all of those who think they have the key,
Realize it's nothing I have done, but rather the
Savior inside of me.
Being obedient, trying to pass each test.
All that God asked for is for me to do my best.

For everyone who has suffered, let it be known…
The only reason life is different now, is because I let God
sit on the thrown.

Even though I had God in my life and was doing better, I still struggled with depression and anxiety. I was untreated and had severe highs and lows. Now, while going to church faithfully, listen to Christian music and doing most things right, I still smoked marijuana.

Addiction still had a hold on me. And it would be years until it let go.

Let's jump ahead a few years. I'm 30. Still untreated for my mental disorder. I had a friend for several years who said he wanted to be more. I asked God to give me love for this man as he was good and kind and served the Lord.

For You

It's me always thinking that I am not good enough for him.
That's exactly how this story begins.
You see I am crazy girl, with insecurities galore.
But there's you, you have always been there to pick my
heart off the floor.

I have lived these past years full of lies,
My love for him I no longer feel the need to disguise.
Years of hoping and hurting, I had left him confused.
I have just been stupid and un-trusting,
afraid of being used.

Now I am ready and all I can see;
Are you now giving up on me.
Can't I just tell him, won't he just see;
that all this time I was too afraid that he
wouldn't love me, for me.

Lots of fighting we have done, and we've had fun too.
But no matter what place we were in we always
stuck like glue!
Its seems as if lately you are drifting further away,
Reach with me, and together we can seize the day.
That line was corny, but I love it still,
Because it's all about His purpose and all about His will.

To not have parted long ago seems odd,
But I am learning to see and understand the will of God.
I think about you daily and pray for you too.
Do you not really know that I want to have
children with you?

I don't say much because you are my friend,
That's important to me and I don't want to see that end.

But I hate you being with other girls, for all this time I thought I
was your world.
I am trusting that what you've said about our future is true.
I don't like any of this but I want to be with you.
You say you don't want to rush, but rush into what -
I love you and you already love me.
We are already here, can't we just be.

I want to go fishing with you and watch the
sun rise at dawn.
I want to clean our house and watch you mow the lawn.
And bast in the pink heavenly glow,
God's grace and love shining down so all may know.
He's here, he's guiding; I hope this is God's timing,
Bringing us both were we need to be,
But please don't give up and please don't stop loving me!

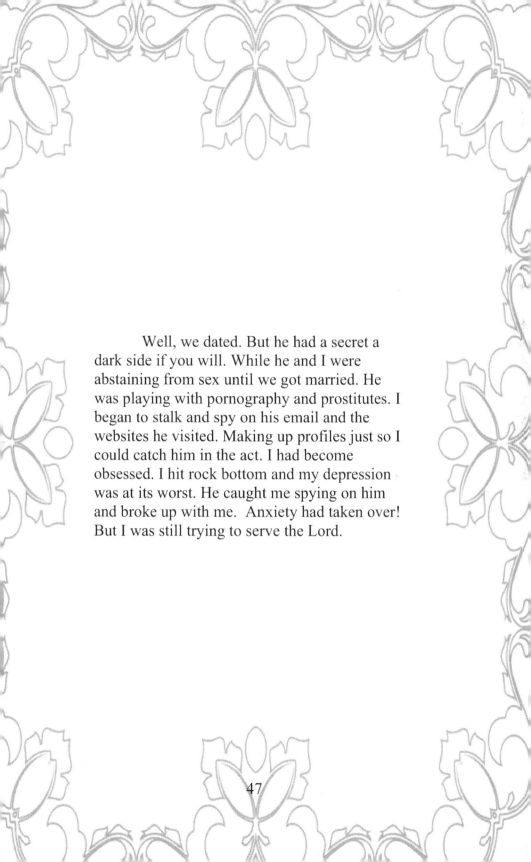

Well, we dated. But he had a secret a dark side if you will. While he and I were abstaining from sex until we got married. He was playing with pornography and prostitutes. I began to stalk and spy on his email and the websites he visited. Making up profiles just so I could catch him in the act. I had become obsessed. I hit rock bottom and my depression was at its worst. He caught me spying on him and broke up with me. Anxiety had taken over! But I was still trying to serve the Lord.

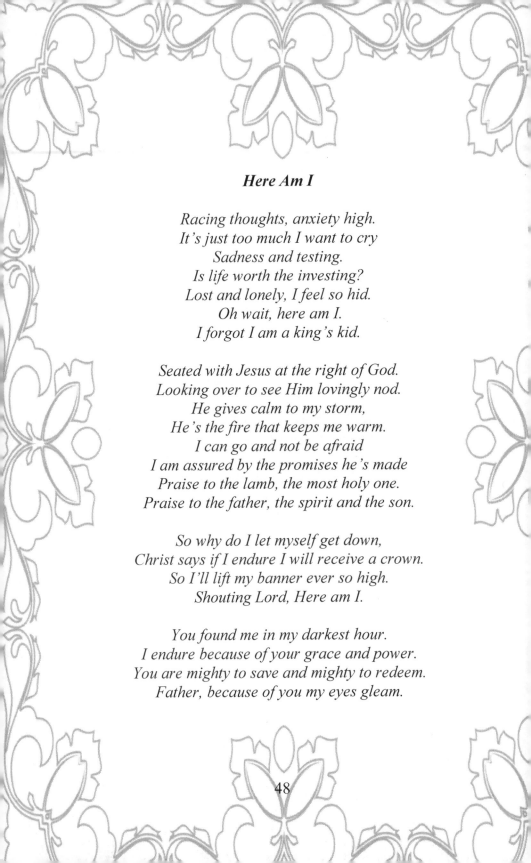

Here Am I

Racing thoughts, anxiety high.
It's just too much I want to cry
Sadness and testing.
Is life worth the investing?
Lost and lonely, I feel so hid.
Oh wait, here am I.
I forgot I am a king's kid.

Seated with Jesus at the right of God.
Looking over to see Him lovingly nod.
He gives calm to my storm,
He's the fire that keeps me warm.
I can go and not be afraid
I am assured by the promises he's made
Praise to the lamb, the most holy one.
Praise to the father, the spirit and the son.

So why do I let myself get down,
Christ says if I endure I will receive a crown.
So I'll lift my banner ever so high.
Shouting Lord, Here am I.

You found me in my darkest hour.
I endure because of your grace and power.
You are mighty to save and mighty to redeem.
Father, because of you my eyes gleam.

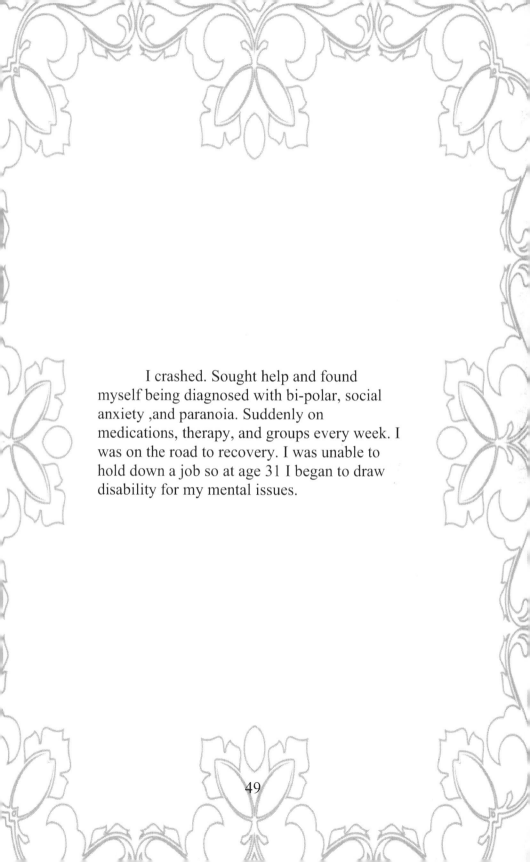

I crashed. Sought help and found myself being diagnosed with bi-polar, social anxiety ,and paranoia. Suddenly on medications, therapy, and groups every week. I was on the road to recovery. I was unable to hold down a job so at age 31 I began to draw disability for my mental issues.

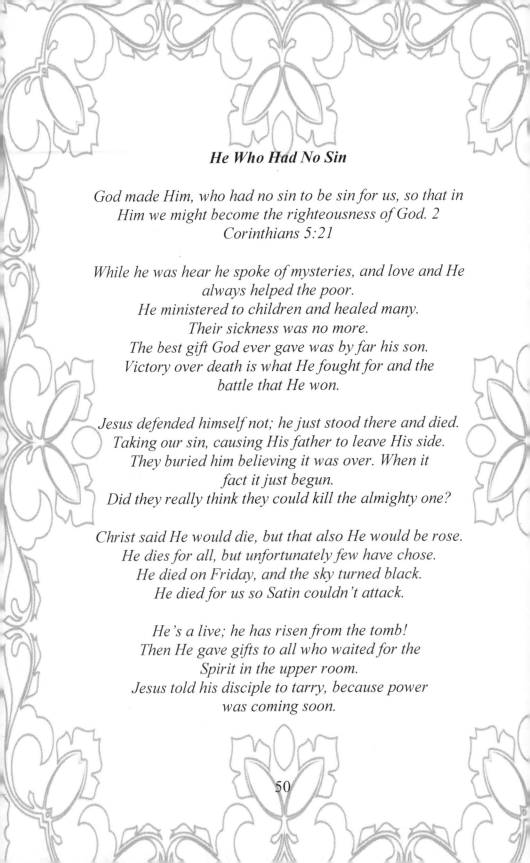

He Who Had No Sin

God made Him, who had no sin to be sin for us, so that in
Him we might become the righteousness of God. 2
Corinthians 5:21

While he was hear he spoke of mysteries, and love and He
always helped the poor.
He ministered to children and healed many.
Their sickness was no more.
The best gift God ever gave was by far his son.
Victory over death is what He fought for and the
battle that He won.

Jesus defended himself not; he just stood there and died.
Taking our sin, causing His father to leave His side.
They buried him believing it was over. When it
fact it just begun.
Did they really think they could kill the almighty one?

Christ said He would die, but that also He would be rose.
He dies for all, but unfortunately few have chose.
He died on Friday, and the sky turned black.
He died for us so Satin couldn't attack.

He's a live; he has risen from the tomb!
Then He gave gifts to all who waited for the
Spirit in the upper room.
Jesus told his disciple to tarry, because power
was coming soon.

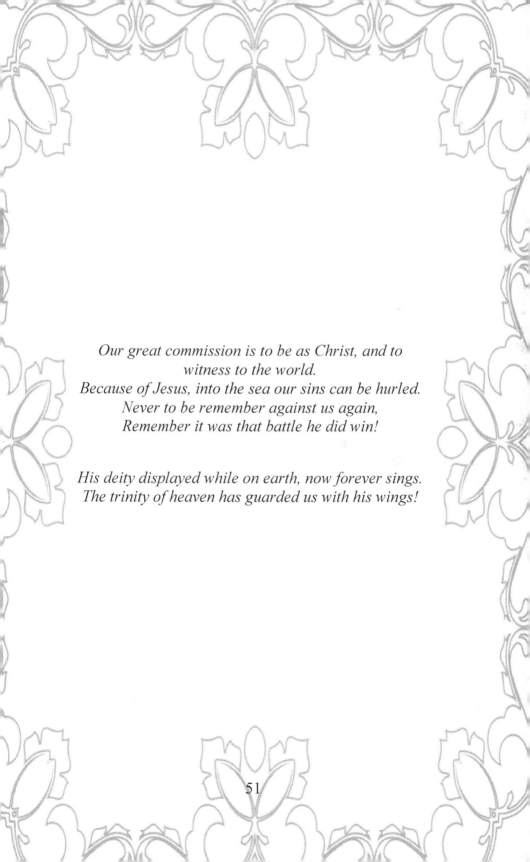

*Our great commission is to be as Christ, and to
witness to the world.
Because of Jesus, into the sea our sins can be hurled.
Never to be remember against us again,
Remember it was that battle he did win!*

*His deity displayed while on earth, now forever sings.
The trinity of heaven has guarded us with his wings!*

Next I bought a house in Coopersville, Michigan. I lived there for five years. During that time, my Aunt Elaine Eaves died. Her funeral was on my birthday. That birthday really sucked. I loved her so very much and was very close to her. They called her Lady

Lady Love

Short and spunky, full of fight.
Being a lady like that, thank God she had His light.
Bold, mighty and fervent in prayer.
Taking on satin, boy did she dare!

She was faithful, she was lady love.
Now she's with our Savior looking down from above.
So much for not eating partially hydrogenated oils, and
taking all those pills.
Because God takes us home not when we are
ready but as He wills.

I will miss her jewelry and those red hats,
The way she teased my daddy and told stories of her cats.
Your eggs at breakfast and your monkey bread too,
Oh Aunt Elaine, There are so many things
that I will miss about you.

If you are listening now I would just like to say,
Thank you for being faithful and for help
in lighting the way.
I know you re at peace now, and your lottery
ticket cashed in;
You are in heaven now; I think it's safe to say "you win!"

What a wonderful day in glory, when Jesus you got to see.
Please say hello to Him and give Him an Eve for me!

In memory of Norma Elaine Eaves Born May 25th, 1945,
gone to be with the Lord Monday October 10th, 2005
(10-12-2005)

53

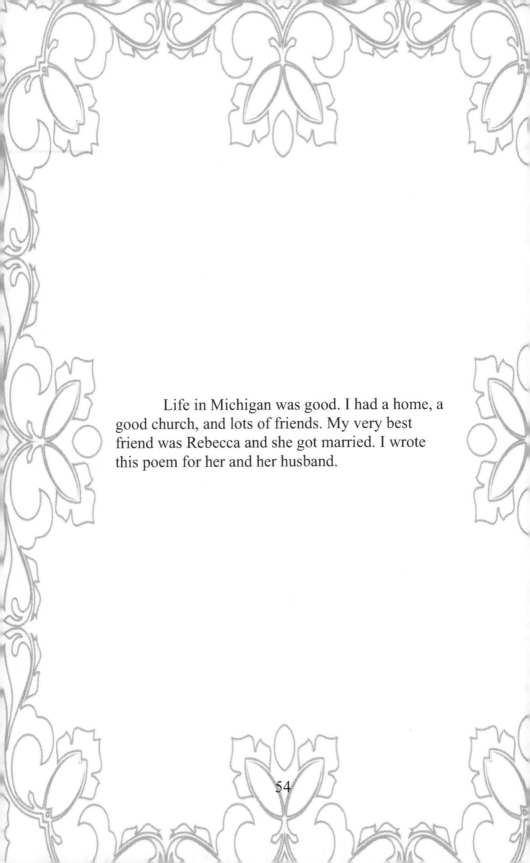

Life in Michigan was good. I had a home, a good church, and lots of friends. My very best friend was Rebecca and she got married. I wrote this poem for her and her husband.

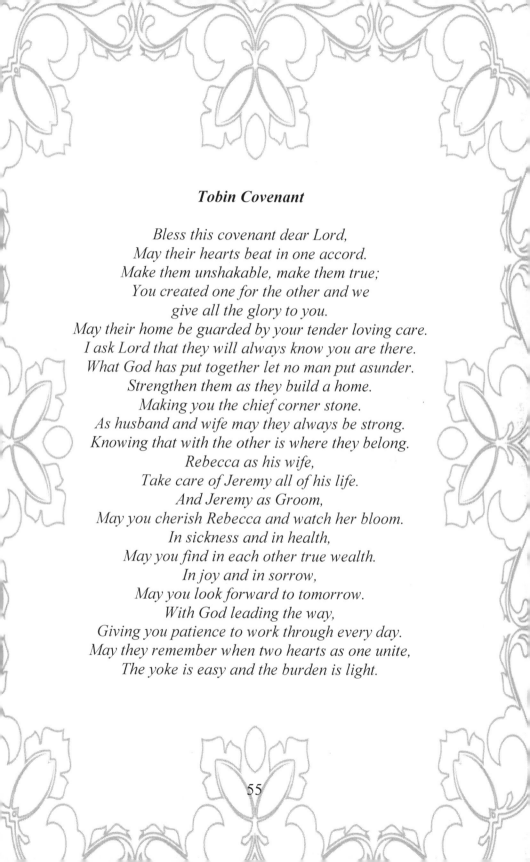

Tobin Covenant

Bless this covenant dear Lord,
May their hearts beat in one accord.
Make them unshakable, make them true;
You created one for the other and we
give all the glory to you.
May their home be guarded by your tender loving care.
I ask Lord that they will always know you are there.
What God has put together let no man put asunder.
Strengthen them as they build a home.
Making you the chief corner stone.
As husband and wife may they always be strong.
Knowing that with the other is where they belong.
Rebecca as his wife,
Take care of Jeremy all of his life.
And Jeremy as Groom,
May you cherish Rebecca and watch her bloom.
In sickness and in health,
May you find in each other true wealth.
In joy and in sorrow,
May you look forward to tomorrow.
With God leading the way,
Giving you patience to work through every day.
May they remember when two hearts as one unite,
The yoke is easy and the burden is light.

One day my folks decided to move to Missouri to retire and I didn't want to be left behind. So I followed. I found Missouri very different. I missed my friends and my church. Of course I found a new church home but it was much bigger and just not the same. So I started looking for friends and since I no longer had my drug dealer I had to find a new one of those too. I was very depressed in and out of the mental hospital. Dating wrong guy after wrong guy. I had begun a life of promiscuity again and I started drinking again.

I found a new man, moved him in with me, behind my parents back. He was an alcoholic and a mean one at that. He hit and talked down to me all the time. Finally I grew tired of is beatings and called the police.

He was arrested and sent to prison. I was tormented in knowing that I had sent someone to prison again and if I had just said the right things or acted the right way, he wouldn't have had to hit me. And he'd be here with me. LIES LIES LIES of the devil! But I allowed them to consume me.

Some time passed and life got worse and I found more wrong friends. I just couldn't take it anymore. On a Wednesday my folks and I went out to eat and I remember sitting there with tears rolling down my cheek, because I just wanted to die.

I went home and took 30 Klonopin, 24 Trazadone's, 9 Vicodin, and what was left of my other prescribed meds and decided to end it all.

Next thing I know I'm in an ambulance headed to the hospital. My folks found me. I was in ICU for a few days and then in the mental ward for almost 2 weeks. This brings us to the beginning of my book.

I'm at the Dorcas House living and fighting for my life. It was such a culture shock to be living with so many different types of people. But it's here that God began to create something new in me.

56

What Does Jesus See in Me?

Sometimes I wonder what He sees in me; really,
What do I have to offer the king?
Then I remember He loves me, praises to Him will I sing.
He has set me free, by covering me with grace,
Oh how I long to see my saviors face.

Again I feel unworthy and I am certainly untrue,
But Jesus loves me in spite of what I do.

He has promised as I confess He will cast my sins away,
So I strive to be more like Him each and every day.

I've heard before that grace is getting what
you don't deserve;
And mercy is not getting what you do.
Let me tell you, I am living proof that's true!

As a human, I seem to focus on my strife.
But God reminds me that He has a plan for my life.

It's a trick of the devil to make us feel so low,
He does not want us to remember, what our
spirit already knows.

So I guess I know what Jesus sees in me,
He is making me, like Him...
No greater thing could there be!

Trust Me

In times of hurting. In times of need.
Turn to our Savior, He's our comfort indeed.
When life brings questions of why,
Remember that it's ok to cry.
God had a plan, just wait and see.
He says my child trust in and relies on me.

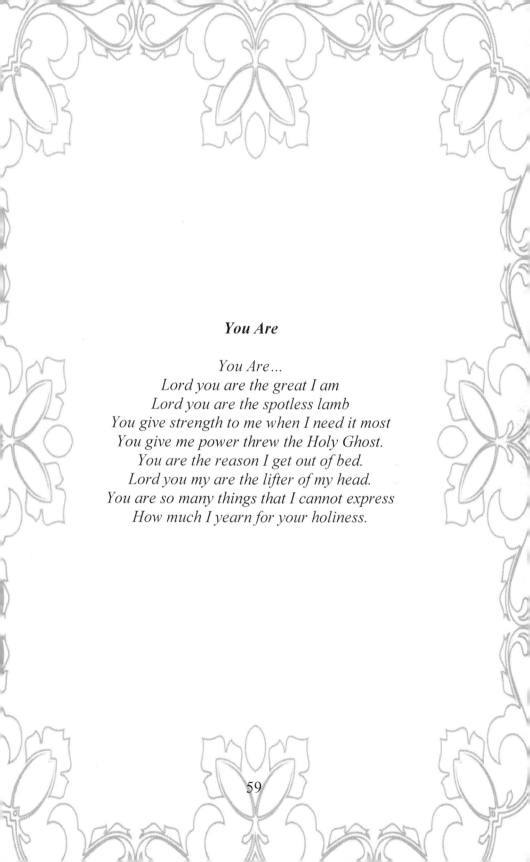

You Are

You Are…
Lord you are the great I am
Lord you are the spotless lamb
You give strength to me when I need it most
You give me power threw the Holy Ghost.
You are the reason I get out of bed.
Lord you my are the lifter of my head.
You are so many things that I cannot express
How much I yearn for your holiness.

Repentant Heart

What a tangled mess we weave,
Causing the Fathers heart to grieve.
Lord please forgive me of my sin.
Come and make me whole again.
Oh gentle one keep me humble,
And guard my steps that I may not stumble.
Give me your heart, your ears, your sight.
Keep me in thy way, guide me day and night.
Break my heart for what breaks yours.
I pray we be in one accord.

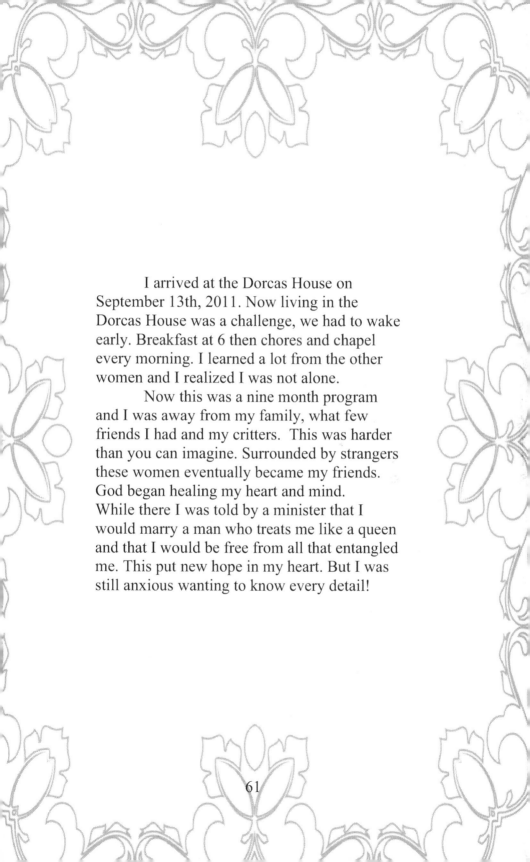

I arrived at the Dorcas House on September 13th, 2011. Now living in the Dorcas House was a challenge, we had to wake early. Breakfast at 6 then chores and chapel every morning. I learned a lot from the other women and I realized I was not alone.

Now this was a nine month program and I was away from my family, what few friends I had and my critters. This was harder than you can imagine. Surrounded by strangers these women eventually became my friends. God began healing my heart and mind. While there I was told by a minister that I would marry a man who treats me like a queen and that I would be free from all that entangled me. This put new hope in my heart. But I was still anxious wanting to know every detail!

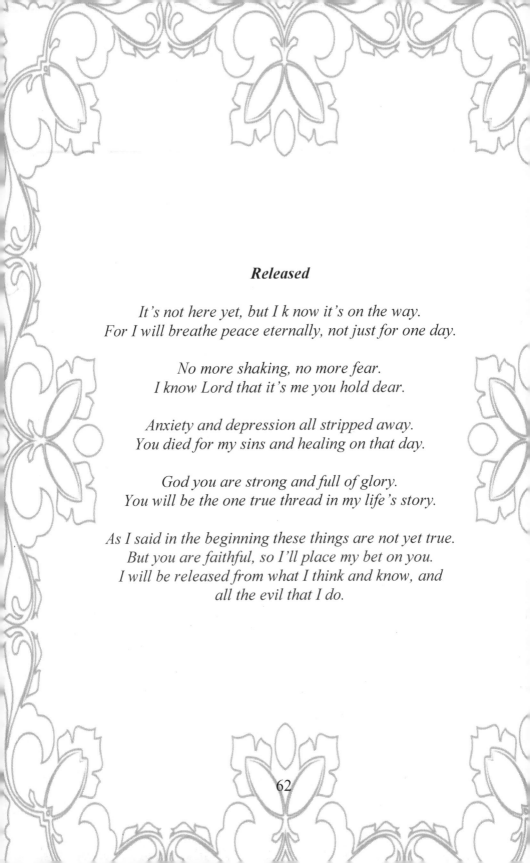

Released

It's not here yet, but I k now it's on the way.
For I will breathe peace eternally, not just for one day.

No more shaking, no more fear.
I know Lord that it's me you hold dear.

Anxiety and depression all stripped away.
You died for my sins and healing on that day.

God you are strong and full of glory.
You will be the one true thread in my life's story.

As I said in the beginning these things are not yet true.
But you are faithful, so I'll place my bet on you.
I will be released from what I think and know, and
all the evil that I do.

If I'm too Busy Freaking

God hasn't even revealed His plan yet,
But here I am worrying and starting to sweat.

Take one day at a time, this much I know.
What He desires for me, He will give and show.

Remember the steps of the righteous are ordered by the
Lord. So why am I stressing and getting all up tight.
His way is perfect, not hidden in darkness, but
full of light.

Oh you silly child of grace.
He will help you find your place.
Just stay calm, always seeking His face.

Here a little, there a little, line upon line.
I just need to remember His plan is divine

Relax, chill out and just go slow
If I'm too busy freaking His plan I will not know.

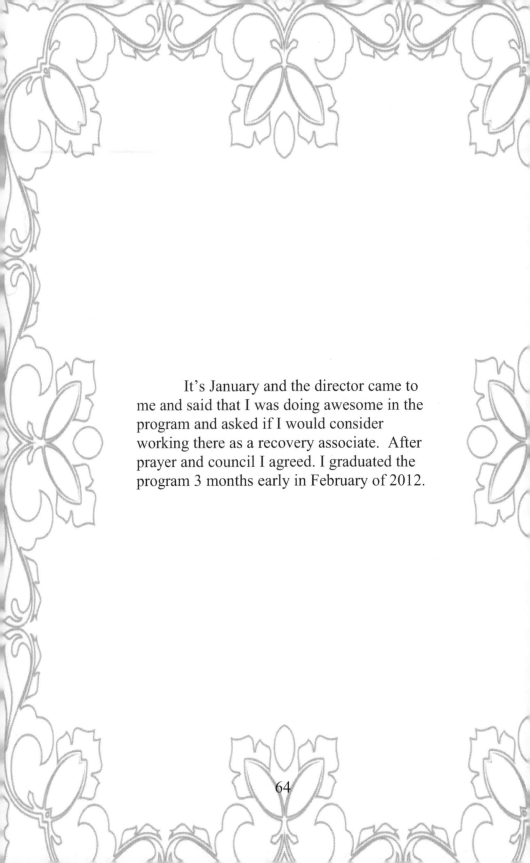

It's January and the director came to me and said that I was doing awesome in the program and asked if I would consider working there as a recovery associate. After prayer and council I agreed. I graduated the program 3 months early in February of 2012.

Graduation Poem

I was raised in a Godly home, dedicated to Him from birth.
But Satan lied to me and so I doubted my worth.

Childhood abuse led to drugs, drinking and lack of self-control.
More than anything I wanted to be made whole.

Dropping out of school, losing all my jobs.
Deep in depression all my family heard were sobs.

I ended up here because of sin in my life.
I caused my own chaos, I caused my own strife.

Down this road I travel being set free!
The change you see now is Christ in me.

What was an attempt to end my life,
I was buried in pain, sorrow cut like a knife.

God saw fit for me to survive,
Now because of Him I surely thrive.

Recovery started out slowly, the light being dim;
You see God had to change the monster I created within.

Disobedience always leads to death.
I was living a lie with every single breath.

Depression and madness, oh such a mess.
But look at me now I stand whole and blessed.

He healed me from depression, set me free from sin.
On this path I journey, I'm living again!

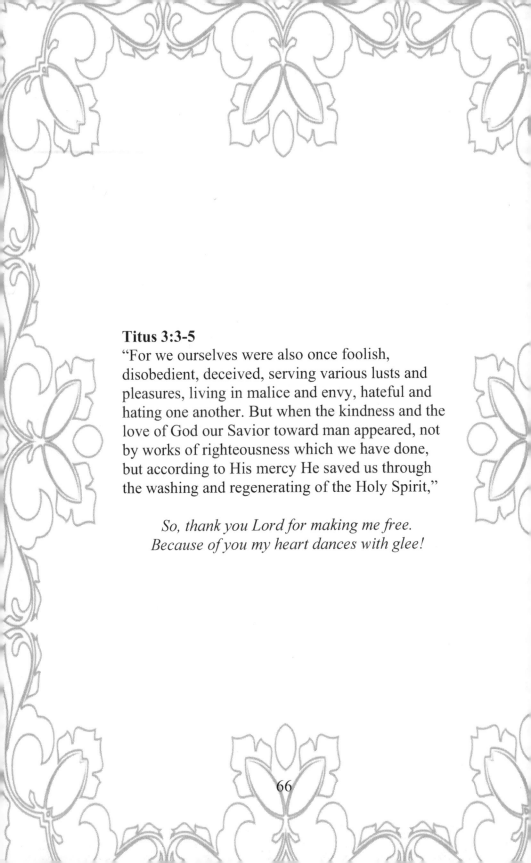

Titus 3:3-5

"For we ourselves were also once foolish, disobedient, deceived, serving various lusts and pleasures, living in malice and envy, hateful and hating one another. But when the kindness and the love of God our Savior toward man appeared, not by works of righteousness which we have done, but according to His mercy He saved us through the washing and regenerating of the Holy Spirit,"

So, thank you Lord for making me free.
Because of you my heart dances with glee!

I graduated February 26, 2012 and began working for the Dorcas House. I took a Christian counseling course at Agape Bible College, I studied for and learned for about 20 hours a week and worked with the residents there for the other 20 hours a week. I gave them guidance and prayed with them and organized outings. But I was still living at the Dorcas House. So I began to look for a place to call my home.

I lived at the Dorcas house until June of 2012. Ten months total! When I found the perfect place for me to live, in a smaller city very near Little Rock. I purchased it and moved in.

I found a great church right across the interstate from my new home and began to get settled in. But it wasn't long until boredom and loneliness set in. When I was going to find this man "who would treat me like a queen?"

Being out of the controlled environment really took its toll on me. Just 2 months after permanently moving to Arkansas, I quit my job at the Dorcas house. I found the 40 hours a week too much to handle.

I started smoking cigarettes again, and even the occasional drink. I decided to get a job at a local gas station. I was tempted and failed. I became very promiscuous and found myself back where God had taken me from.

Once again I was depressed in and out of the hospital for suicidal tendencies. I finally started a day treatment program for mentally ill people. I was coping. I finally lost my job at the gas station due to missed work. I was devastated. I began smoking marijuana again to help with the pain of my sorrow.

Now you may remember I told you I had 3 cats and a dog? Well while living in the Dorcas house 2 of my cats had to be put down and the other my vet found a good home for. But I still had my dog, Lewis! Whom I loved very much and he was my best friend for 10 years. So after only having him back for 6 months, he became very ill and I had to put him down.

I couldn't breathe. I was so depressed. My whole word was shaken.

For Lewis

It's so strange without you here.
I want you close. I wish I could hold you near.
You playing with your squeak squeak and running
down the hall.
You were the best dog ever, the best dog of all.
I miss the way you'd wag your butt.
You were a strange breed but the perfect mutt.
Your broke ear and Maybelline eyes.
I believe your waiting for me up in the skies.
You were a Christian dog; you loved to praise the Lord.
I tried to give you the very best, all that I could afford.
I miss you sitting shot gun when we'd go to a ride.
I just plain miss you. I wish you were by my side.

Then I meet a man at the day treatment facility. His name is Jeff .He was and is a great guy. We began to date and we very quickly fell in love. He was a recovering addict. One who had only recently given his life to Christ. I was and was not a good influence on him. I brought him to church with me and very soon God started to change him. And by doing so, God changed me.

He proposed on October 9th, 2013. And I said yes! We were married the following year in May of 2014. And yes folks, he treats me like a queen! God kept his promise as he always does. Thank you God for being true to your word!

So now we are at the present, 2015! While I am still medicated for bi-polar and anxiety I no longer smoke marijuana and haven't for a year and a half! And I do face depression at times but I just speak Gods word that I am an over comer! And you can be too!

My book is entitled RELEASED~ Healing Through Bi-Polar because God gets me through my mental disorder.

And while I have not been totally healed, I am being healed every day. I just have to walk in faith so that I may receive all that He has given.

While sharing these details of my life can be embarrassing, I have learned that I have the chance to help others along their journey and that I must be inside out...

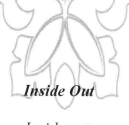

Inside Out

Inside out,
That's what serving Jesus is all about.

What you hide bring to light.
You will see He is merciful yet full of might.
Righting every wrong,
Let His salvation be your song.

In His image you are made.
So stand firm and do not be afraid.
Afraid to wear your heart on your sleeve.
To show others what you have grieved.

Let your life be a song,
That to Jesus you now belong.
Speak with integrity, speak with truth.
You can forget the shame of your youth.

May your test be a testimony,
That you stand for Christ only.
Speak of what He does,
By this encourage others and show them His love.

He is beautiful and full of grace.
Seek you master's face.
Serve the Lord with all you heart;
Of His inheritance you are a part.

So, let your inside out!
Because that's what serving Jesus is all about!

If you'd like to be free. To experience the Joy and peace that I now have. All you must do is say a prayer and ask Jesus into your heart and to forgive you of all your sins. And He will come in and cleanse you and start changing you. Life won't be easy, but He will get you through!

If you said that prayer I encourage you to find a good church, one who teaches the Word, pray, get and read the Bible daily.

BE BLESSED and I'll be praying for you!

Katrina

Made in the USA
Columbia, SC
01 August 2018